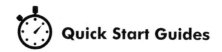
Quick Start Guides

The Essential
INTERMITTENT
FASTING DIET
Cookbook

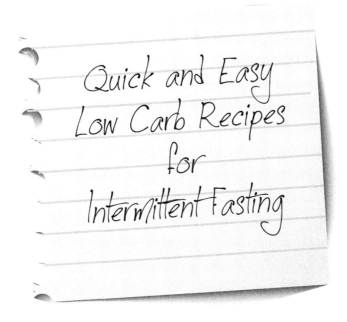

Quick and Easy Low Carb Recipes for Intermittent Fasting

5:2 & 16:8 Diet Friendly
Delicious Calorie-Counted Recipes

First published in 2020 by Erin Rose Publishing

Text and illustration copyright © 2020 Erin Rose Publishing

Design: Julie Anson

ISBN: 978-1-9161523-7-3

A CIP record for this book is available from the British Library.

DISCLAIMER: This book is for informational purposes only and not intended as a substitute for the medical advice, diagnosis or treatment of a physician or qualified healthcare provider. The reader should consult a physician before undertaking a new health care regime and in all matters relating to his/her health, and particularly with respect to any symptoms that may require diagnosis or medical attention.

While every care has been taken in compiling the recipes for this book we cannot accept responsibility for any problems which arise as a result of preparing one of the recipes. The author and publisher disclaim responsibility for any adverse effects that may arise from the use or application of the recipes in this book. Some of the recipes in this book include nuts. If you have a nut allergy it's important to avoid these.

CONTENTS

INTRODUCTION

If you are ready to lose weight quickly and sustainably, Intermittent Fasting (IF) could be for you. So, whether you are following the 5:2 diet, the 16:8 diet, or Time Restricted Eating, this easy-to-use cookbook provides you with delicious recipes to make losing weight with intermittent fasting easy.

This **Quick Start Guide** provides you with plenty of calorie-counted, low-carb recipes which help you to feel fuller for longer, reduce food cravings and prevent you from over-eating when you break your fast. You can enjoy simple, tasty recipes and achieve great results with whichever fasting program works for you. This handy cookbook gives you food options for meals, snacks and treats which will make fasting times easier with satisfying, easy and delicious food to look forward to.

This intermittent fasting recipe book contains lovely calorie-counted recipes and gives you the essential information and tips for fast weight loss with simple, great-tasting, recipes to optimise health and well-being. Eating the right food during feasting times is essential to preventing hunger, losing weight and improving your health.

The rise in the popularity of fasting is founded on good, sustainable results, backed by research showing healthy weight loss, plus other benefits such as mood improvement, vitality and longevity.

With intermittent fasting you eat food only in a specific time window and fast the rest of the time. During your eating window, you can enjoy plenty of protein, healthy fats and vegetables which will help you feel satisfied and prevent hunger pangs.

Whether you are looking for food ideas when following the 5:2 diet, 16:8 diet, time restricted eating calorie restriction or building up to the warrior diet, there are plenty of recipes to help you achieve your weight loss goals.

Are you ready to start improving your health and wellbeing? Let's get started!

What Can Intermittent Fasting Do For You?

Intermittent fasting on the 5:2 diet has been a great success where many have achieved their weight loss goals by fasting 2 days a week. Intermittent fasting can be tailored to suit you and by using time restricted eating you eat only during a certain window of time. Your fasting window can be 12, 16 or 20 hours a day, involving stretching the overnight fasting period, so you would consume no calories during this time. They key is to listen to your body and do what works best for you.

Fasting allows your body to detoxify, heal, grow and repair. You can start with a shorter fasting time and gradually increase it. Doing the 16:8 fast is a popular choice, involving fasting for 16 hours and only eating during an 8 hour period. So, if for example, you began fasting at 7pm you could begin eating again at 11am. Avoid eating late in the evening as your body has less need for fuel while you sleep.

Research has shown the benefits of intermittent fasting include improved cognitive function, healthier blood pressure, better cholesterol and sustainable weight loss in those who may have had difficulty losing weight, especially if it's linked to metabolic syndrome. Research is still continuing, and so far the results look great. Studies have found intermittent fasting is not only excellent for weight loss and reducing belly fat, but for reducing insulin resistance, improving blood sugar and protecting the body from type 2 diabetes.

Fasting and eating low carbohydrate foods during your eating time, can help you achieve ketosis. This is a natural metabolic process where the body switches to fat burning mode instead of using glucose.

So avoiding starchy carbohydrates when you are intermittent fasting will help curb your appetite and increase weight loss, plus many people feel lighter and brighter too.

The benefits of intermittent fasting are more than just losing extra weight and it's suitable for most people who have extra pounds to lose. However, check with your doctor or health care professional that it is safe for you begin intermittent fasting before you begin.

Getting Started

Beginning any diet can be daunting so allow yourself to do it in whatever way works best for you.

Decide what type of fasting is best for you depending on how much weight you want to lose and what fits in with your lifestyle. You can choose fast days for example as in the 5:2 diet, or 16:8 hours or another time restricted eating pattern. Basically tailor it to suit you and you may find you can increase your fasting time.

During eating periods, you can also restrict calories or eat sensibly during this time.

You can also choose to eat with time restrictions on non-fasting days with time restricted eating, for instance eating only within an 8-12 hour window.

Plan which days you are fasting so you can be prepared. Increase your water intake to help the body eliminate fat.

You can choose to extend your overnight fast and have a late brunch followed by an early evening meal, or you could have lunch and dinner or opt for 3 lighter meals a day. This may take a little experimenting and developing as you figure out what works best for you.

Remember that avoiding starchy carbohydrates, refined carbs, grains and sugars, will help balance blood sugar and reduce hunger pangs. Make sure you eat plenty of vegetables, proteins and healthy fats.

Fasting allows your body to burn fat, so don't be tempted to snack during this time and remember this includes drinks other than water, especially milky or sugary drinks and alcohol.

You can gradually begin intermittent fasting and increase your fasting time. For instance, you could limit yourself to only eating in a 12 hour time period, say 7pm to 7am and increase fasting time by eating only in an 8 hour window, say 10am until 6pm or you could increase it further. Always listen to your body and avoid eating before bedtime. As your body adapts you may find you have more energy and reduced hunger and feel ready to extend your fast further.

This cookbook also contains recipes for healthy, low-carb desserts, however these should only be eaten in moderation and avoid them completely if you have sugar cravings or hunger pangs. These can be reduced or eliminated completely by avoiding sugar and starchy carbohydrates.

Fasting is not suitable for the elderly, convalescing, children, during pregnancy or breastfeeding, or if you suffer from or have a history of an eating disorder or have a low BMI or have other medical conditions. Always seek your doctor's advice and especially regarding medication changes.

Diet Tips

- Keep a food diary. Writing down what you eat helps you track your calorie consumption and you can also log how you are feeling including energy, sleep, weight loss and fluid intake. It's great to reflect and see how you're doing.

- On non-fasting days, don't binge. You can stick to the low carb recipes and don't over-do the portions.

- You can fill up on high volume foods like broccoli, cauliflower, carrots and heaps of lettuce or spinach without adding large amounts of carbohydrates.

- At mealtimes, replace starchy carbohydrates with lots of veggies and you'll feel less sluggish and hungry.

- Schedule in easy meals and plan them in advance so you avoid temptation. That way you can also avoid missing a meal.

- Always drink plenty of water!

- You may experience headaches in the first couple of days as your body adjusts. Relax as much as possible and remember to drink plenty of water. You will need extra fluid as your body burns off excess fat and you shed those extra pounds.

If you get sugar cravings, they will pass! Once your body switches to burning fat for fuel it will be easier.

SMOOTHIES

Iced Coffee Smoothie

**SERVES
1**

152
calories
per serving

Ingredients

1 teaspoon instant coffee

½ avocado, stone removed and peeled

200mls (7fl oz) almond milk

A few ice cubes

Method

Place all of the ingredients into a blender and process until smooth and creamy. You can add crushed ice after processing if your blender doesn't tolerate ice cubes.

Chocolate Nut Butter Smoothie

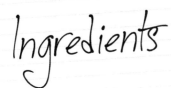

Ingredients

2 teaspoons 100% cocoa powder

1 small banana, peeled

2 teaspoons smooth peanut butter

200mls (7fl oz) almond milk

Small handful of ice cubes

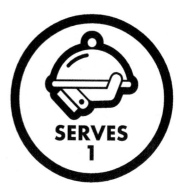

SERVES 1

227 calories per serving

Method

Place all of the ingredients into a blender and process until smooth. You can add crushed ice after blending if you'd prefer. Serve and drink straight away.

Mint Avocado Smoothie

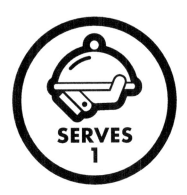

SERVES 1

348
calories
per serving

Ingredients

250mls (8fl oz) almond milk

8 fresh mint leaves

1 avocado, stone and skin removed

Juice of ½ lime

Method

Place the ingredients into a blender and blitz until smooth. You can add extra almond milk or some water if you like it thinner.

Red Berry Refresher

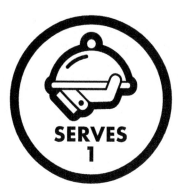

SERVES 1

95 calories per serving

Ingredients

100g (3½ oz) mixed berries: strawberries, blueberries, raspberries and blackberries

1 carrot, peeled

25mls (1fl oz) coconut milk

Juice of ½ a lime

Method

Place all the ingredients into a blender and add just enough water to cover the ingredients. Blitz until smooth and creamy.

Cashew & Apricot Smoothie

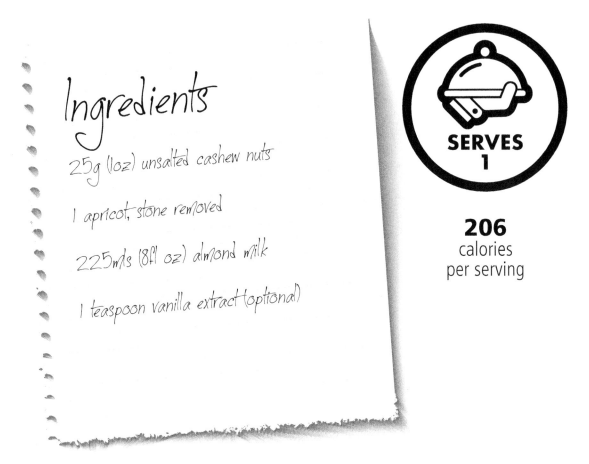

Ingredients

25g (1oz) unsalted cashew nuts

1 apricot, stone removed

225mls (8fl oz) almond milk

1 teaspoon vanilla extract (optional)

SERVES 1

206 calories per serving

Method

Place all of the ingredients into a blender and process until smooth. Serve and drink straight away.

Apple & Cucumber Smoothie

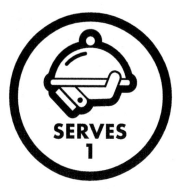

SERVES 1

87
calories
per serving

Ingredients

½ cucumber, roughly chopped

1 green apple, cored

Juice of ½ lemon

Method

Place the ingredients into a blender and top up with just enough water to cover them.
Blitz until smooth. Serve and drink straight away.

Golden Turmeric Smoothie

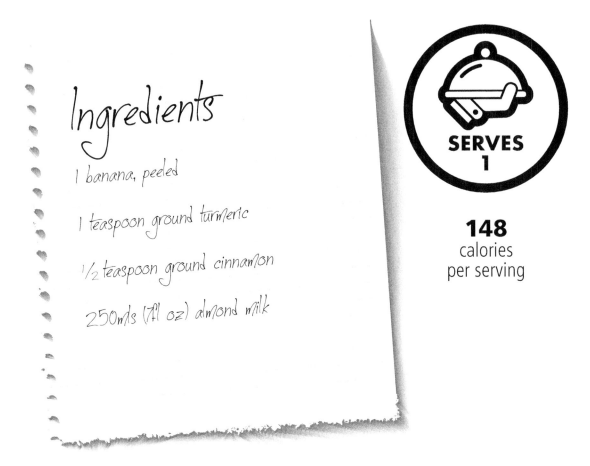

Ingredients

1 banana, peeled

1 teaspoon ground turmeric

½ teaspoon ground cinnamon

250mls (7fl oz) almond milk

SERVES 1

148 calories per serving

Method

Place all of the ingredients into a blender and process until smooth. Serve and drink straight away.

Creamy Orange & Melon Smoothie

Ingredients

50g (2oz) plain Greek yogurt

1 medium orange, peeled

1 pear, cored

½ honeydew melon, flesh only

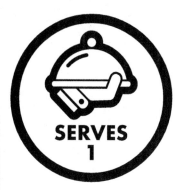

SERVES 1

144 calories per serving

Method

Place all of the ingredients into a blender and add just enough water to cover them. Blitz until smooth. Pour and enjoy!

Cherry & Raspberry Smoothie

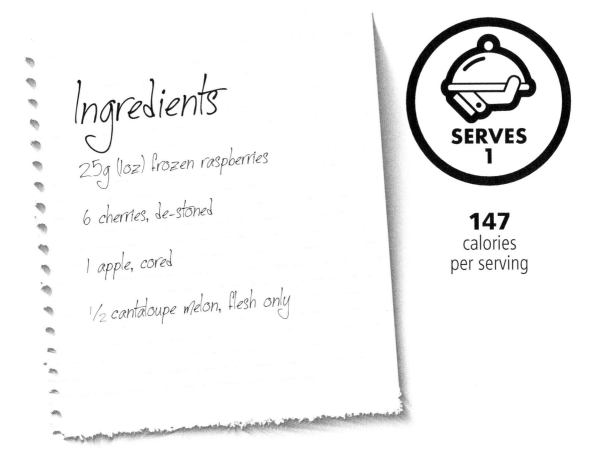

Ingredients

25g (1oz) frozen raspberries

6 cherries, de-stoned

1 apple, cored

1/2 cantaloupe melon, flesh only

SERVES 1

147 calories per serving

Method

Place all the ingredients into a blender and add just enough water to cover the ingredients. Blitz until smooth. Serve and drink straight away.

Coconut, Lime & Lettuce Smoothie

Ingredients

1 handful of fresh lettuce leaves

1 apple, cored

1/4 cucumber

Juice of 1/2 lime

225mls (7fl oz) chilled coconut water

SERVES 1

116 calories per serving

Method

Place all of the ingredients into a blender and blitz until smooth. Serve straight away.

LIGHT
MEALS

Sausage & Egg Bake

Ingredients

100g (3½ oz) Cheddar cheese, grated (shredded)
50g (2oz) fresh spinach leaves
8 thin sausages
8 eggs, beaten
3 large tomatoes, roughly chopped
1 onion, chopped
2 teaspoon fresh parsley
1 teaspoon paprika
1 tablespoon olive oil

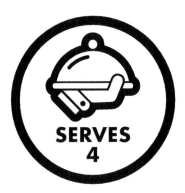

SERVES 4

411 calories per serving

Method

Heat the olive oil in a frying pan, add the sausages and onion into the pan and fry until the sausages are completely cooked. Transfer the sausages and onion to an ovenproof dish. Add in the tomatoes, spinach leaves, eggs, parsley and paprika and mix well. Scatter the grated cheese over the top. Transfer the dish to the oven and bake at 200C/400F for around 35 minutes until the mixture is completely firm.

Savoury Muffins

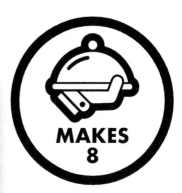

MAKES 8

138
calories
per serving

Ingredients

200g (7oz) ham, chopped

75g (3oz) Cheddar cheese, grated (shredded)

8 large eggs, beaten

1 red pepper (bell pepper), finely chopped

1 small courgette (zucchini), finely chopped

Method

Combine the beaten eggs with the ham, cheese, red pepper (bell pepper) and courgette (zucchini). Place paper cases inside a 8–hole muffin tin. Spoon the egg mixture into the cases. Transfer them to the oven and bake at 180C/360F for 20 minutes or until the eggs are completely set. These are so appealing and easy to make. They can be eaten hot or cold. You can try a variety of fillings and make good use of leftovers, such as chicken, prawns, beef or roast vegetables.

Keto Bread

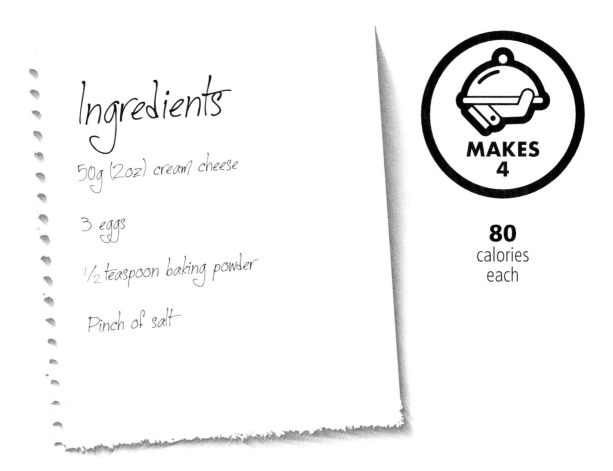

Ingredients

50g (2oz) cream cheese

3 eggs

½ teaspoon baking powder

Pinch of salt

**MAKES
4**

80
calories
each

Method

Line two baking trays with greaseproof paper. Separate the egg yolks from the whites and place them in separate bowls. Add the cream cheese and a pinch of salt to the egg yolks and mix to a smooth batter. In the other bowl, add the baking powder to the egg whites and beat them until they form stiff peaks. Fold the egg yolk mixture into the beaten egg whites and gently combine. Scoop out a large spoonful of the mixture to form a round shape. Transfer them to the oven and bake at 150C/300F for 15-20 minutes until golden. Allow them to cool then store in a plastic bag until ready to use. These delicious bready rolls are a delicious alternative to sandwiches.

Choc & Nut Low Carb Muesli

Ingredients

SERVES 1

374 calories per serving

1 tablespoon chopped hazelnuts

1 tablespoon flaxseeds (linseeds)

1 tablespoon desiccated (shredded) coconut

1 teaspoon sunflower seeds

1 teaspoon pumpkin seeds

1 teaspoon cacao nibs

1/4 teaspoon stevia sweetener (optional)

75mls (3fl oz) almond milk

Method

Place the nuts, seeds, cacao nibs and sweetener (if using) into a bowl and pour the milk on top. Eat straight away.

Cheese & Spinach Slice

Ingredients

225g (8oz) mozzarella cheese, grated (shredded)

120g (4oz) ground almonds

25g (1oz) fresh spinach leaves, chopped

2 eggs

1 onion, finely chopped

1 teaspoon baking powder

200mls (7fl oz) almond milk

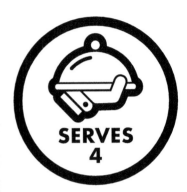

SERVES 4

390 calories per serving

Method

Place the spinach into a saucepan, cover it with warm water, bring it to the boil and cook for 3 minutes. Drain it and set aside. Place the ground almonds in a bowl and add in the eggs, milk and baking powder and mix well. Add in the chopped onion, spinach and cheese and combine the mixture. Spoon the mixture into an ovenproof dish and smooth it out. Transfer it to the oven and bake at 190C/375F for 35 minutes. Cut into slices before serving.

Chicken, Avocado & Basil Omelette

Ingredients

25g (1oz) Cheddar cheese, grated (shredded)

50g (2oz) chicken leftovers, chopped

2 eggs, beaten

Flesh of ½ avocado, chopped

1 teaspoon fresh basil

1 teaspoon olive oil

Freshly ground black pepper

**SERVES
1**

491
calories
per serving

Method

Heat the olive oil in a frying pan then pour in the beaten egg mixture. When it begins to set, sprinkle on the cheese, basil, chicken and chopped avocado. Cook until the eggs are completely set and the cheese has melted. Season with black pepper.

Feta Cheese & Courgette Omelette

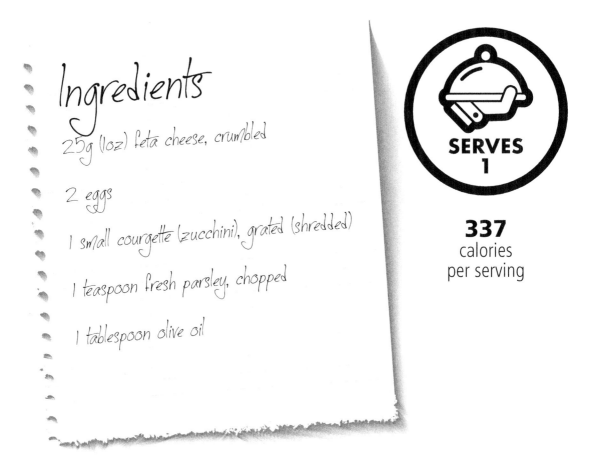

Ingredients

25g (1oz) feta cheese, crumbled

2 eggs

1 small courgette (zucchini), grated (shredded)

1 teaspoon fresh parsley, chopped

1 tablespoon olive oil

SERVES 1

337 calories per serving

Method

Place the eggs in a bowl and whisk them. Stir in the cheese and courgette (zucchini). Heat the olive oil in a frying pan. Pour in the egg mixture and cook until it is set. Sprinkle with parsley and serve.

Mediterranean Omelette

Ingredients

50g (2oz) tinned cannellini beans, drained

50g (2oz) mushrooms, chopped

2 eggs

1 red pepper (bell pepper)

1 tablespoon olive oil

A small handful of fresh basil, chopped

Dash of Tabasco sauce or a sprinkle of chilli powder

SERVES 1

394
calories
per serving

Method

Heat the olive oil in a pan. Add the mushrooms, pepper (bell pepper) and beans. Cook for 3-4 minutes until the vegetables have softened. Remove them and set aside. Whisk the eggs in a bowl and pour them into the pan. Once the eggs begin to set, return the mushrooms, peppers and beans and spread them onto the eggs. Sprinkle with basil, chilli or Tabasco sauce. Serve and eat straight away.

Pizza Style Mug Omelette

Ingredients

25g (1oz) mozzarella cheese

2 cherry tomatoes, chopped

2 eggs

2 teaspoons chopped red pepper (bell pepper)

1/4 teaspoon dried oregano

1/2 teaspoon softened butter

SERVES 1

221
calories
per serving

Method

Crack the eggs into a large mug and beat them. Add in the remaining ingredients. Place the mug in a microwave and cook on full power for 30 seconds. Stir and return it to the microwave for another 30 seconds, stir and cook for another 30-60 seconds or until the egg is set. As a variation try adding cooked sausage, bacon, chicken, chorizo and spring onions (scallions). Or you can simply go for plain eggs as a quick and easy alternative to scrambling.

Thai Chicken Soup

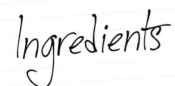

Ingredients

100g (3½ oz) cooked chicken, chopped

½ teaspoon thai red curry paste

½ red pepper (bell pepper), sliced

50mls (2fl oz) coconut milk

200mls (7fl oz) chicken stock (broth)

1 teaspoon fresh coriander (cilantro), chopped

½ teaspoon ground ginger

1 teaspoon olive oil

SERVES
1

297
calories
per serving

Method

Heat the olive oil in a frying pan, add the red pepper (bell pepper) and cook for 3 minutes. Pour in the stock (broth), ginger and add the curry paste. Cook for 1 minute. Pour in the coconut milk and stir in the chicken. Cook for 10-15 minutes. Sprinkle in the coriander (cilantro) and serve.

Tomato & Pesto Soup

Ingredients

3 tomatoes

1 stalk of celery, chopped

1 teaspoon pesto sauce

2 teaspoons crème fraîche

360mls (12fl oz) hot stock (broth)

Freshly ground black pepper

**SERVES
1**

81
calories
per serving

Method

Place the tomatoes, celery and pesto into a saucepan and add the water and stock (broth). Cook for 8-10 minutes. Using a hand blender or food processor blitz the soup until it's smooth. Add the crème fraîche and stir well. Season with salt and pepper then serve.

Quick Chicken & Asparagus Soup

Ingredients

2 asparagus stalks, finely chopped

1 small chicken breast, finely chopped

1 small carrot, finely diced

1/2 small courgette (zucchini), finely chopped

250mls (8fl oz) chicken stock (broth)

1/2 teaspoon lemon juice

1 teaspoon olive oil

Freshly ground black pepper

SERVES 1

235 calories per serving

Method

Heat the olive oil in a saucepan, add the chicken and cook it for 5 minutes, stirring occasionally. Pour in the stock (broth) and add the courgette (zucchini), lemon juice, carrot and asparagus. Bring it to the boil, reduce the heat and simmer for 15 minutes. Season and serve.

Creamy Leek & Ham Soup

Ingredients

4 slices of ham, finely chopped

2 small leeks, chopped

2 cloves of garlic, chopped

1 tablespoon fresh parsley, chopped

2 tablespoons crème fraîche

2 teaspoons butter

1 onion, peeled and chopped

500mls (1 pint) vegetable stock (broth)

SERVES
2

165
calories
per serving

Method

Heat the butter in a saucepan, add the onion, leek and garlic and cook for 5 minutes until they have softened. Add in the stock (broth), bring it to the boil, reduce the heat and simmer for 15 minutes. Stir in the parsley and crème fraîche. Using a food processor or hand blender process the soup until smooth and creamy. Stir in the ham and serve.

Creamy Tomato Soup

Ingredients

2 x 400g (14oz) tins of chopped tomatoes

25g (1oz) butter

1 red onion, chopped

600mls (1 pint) vegetable stock (broth)

150mls (5fl oz) double cream (heavy cream)

2 tablespoons basil, chopped

Sea salt

Freshly ground black pepper

SERVES 4

293
calories
per serving

Method

Heat the butter in a saucepan, add the onion and cook for 5 minutes. Add in the tomatoes and stock (broth) and bring it to the boil. Reduce the heat and simmer for 5 minutes. Using a food processor and or hand blender blitz until smooth. Pour in the cream and warm it. Sprinkle in the basil and season with salt and pepper. Serve straight away.

Green Vegetable Soup

Ingredients

450g (1lb) broccoli, chopped

1 large leek, chopped

1 fennel bulb, chopped

1 courgette (zucchini), chopped

1 handful parsley, chopped

1 handful chives, chopped

Sea salt

Freshly ground black pepper

SERVES 4

61 calories per serving

Method

Place the broccoli, leek, courgette (zucchini) and fennel in enough water to cover them and bring to the boil. Simmer for 10-15 minutes or until the vegetables are tender. Stir in the herbs. Using a hand blender or food processor blend until the soup becomes smooth. Add more water if required to adjust the consistency. Season and serve.

Cream of Asparagus Soup

Ingredients

900g (2lbs) asparagus

2 tablespoons crème fraîche

1 onion, chopped

1 tablespoon olive oil

900mls (1½ pints) chicken stock (broth)

Sea salt

Freshly ground black pepper

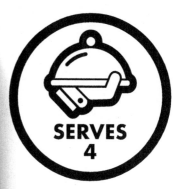

SERVES 4

104 calories per serving

Method

Heat the oil in a large saucepan, add the onion and cook for 5 minutes. Break off the tough root end of the asparagus and roughly chop it. Place it in the saucepan and add the stock (broth). Bring it to the boil, reduce the heat and simmer for 20 minutes. Using a food processor or hand blender, process the soup until smooth and creamy. Stir in the crème fraîche. Season and serve.

Cream Of Mushroom Soup

Ingredients

450g (1lb) mushrooms, chopped

1 large leek, finely chopped

1 tablespoon cornflour (corn starch)

750mls (1½ pints) vegetable stock (broth)

150mls (5fl oz) crème fraîche

1 tablespoon olive oil

Sea salt

Freshly ground black pepper

SERVES 4

126 calories per serving

Method

Heat the olive oil in a saucepan. Add the leek and mushrooms and cook for 8 minutes or until the vegetables are soft. Sprinkle in the cornflour (corn starch) and stir. Pour in the stock (broth), bring it to the boil, cover and simmer for 20 minutes. Stir in the crème fraîche. Using a hand blender or food processor, blend the soup until smooth. Return to the heat if necessary. Season with salt and pepper just before serving.

Quick Bean & Parmesan Soup

Ingredients

100g (3½ oz) cannellini beans, drained
3 spring onions (scallions), chopped
1 tomato, de-seeded and chopped
1 small carrot, finely diced
1 clove of garlic, crushed
½ small courgette (zucchini) finely diced
½ teaspoon dried mixed herbs
1 tablespoon Parmesan cheese, grated (shredded)
1 tablespoon tomato purée (paste)
250mls (8fl oz) vegetable stock (broth)
1 teaspoon olive oil

**SERVES
1**

225
calories
per serving

Method

Heat the olive oil in a saucepan, add the carrots, spring onions (scallions), courgette (zucchini) and garlic. Cook for 4 minutes or until the vegetables have softened. Pour in the stock (broth), mixed herbs and the tomato purée (paste). Bring to the boil, reduce the heat and simmer for 10 minutes. Add the beans and tomatoes and warm them completely. Serve the soup with the Parmesan cheese sprinkled on top. Eat straight away.

Beef & Mushroom Soup

SERVES 1

133
calories
per serving

Ingredients

50g (2oz) cooked sliced beef, chopped

2 large mushrooms, finely sliced

3 spring onions (scallions), finely chopped

1 stick of celery, finely chopped

1 teaspoon olive oil

250mls (8fl oz) beef stock (broth)

Sea salt

Freshly ground black pepper

Method

Heat the oil in a saucepan, add the mushrooms, spring onions (scallions) and celery and cook for 3-4 minutes. Pour in the stock (broth) and chopped beef. Bring it to the boil, reduce the heat and cook for 10 minutes. Season with salt and pepper. Serve and enjoy.

Ham & Lentil Soup

Ingredients

50g (2oz) lentils
2 slices of ham, chopped
2 florets of cauliflower, chopped
2 stalks of celery, chopped
1 clove of garlic, chopped
1 small carrot, chopped
1 tablespoon fresh parsley, chopped
1 small onion, chopped
1 bay leaf
250mls (8fl oz) vegetable stock (broth)
Sea salt
Freshly ground black pepper

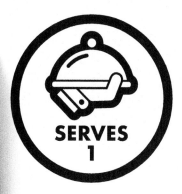

**SERVES
1**

169
calories
per serving

Method

Place all of the ingredients into a saucepan. Bring it to the boil then reduce the heat and simmer for 30 minutes. Remove the bay leaf from the soup. Using a hand blender or food processor blitz the soup until smooth. Season with salt and pepper then serve.

Cream of Red Pepper Soup

Ingredients

1 red pepper (bell pepper), de-seeded and finely chopped

2 teaspoons crème fraîche

250mls (8fl oz) hot stock (broth)

Sea salt

Freshly ground black pepper

SERVES 1

54 calories per serving

Method

Place the red pepper (bell pepper) into a saucepan and pour in the hot stock (broth). Bring the ingredients to the boil, reduce the heat and simmer for a few minutes until the pepper has softened. Using a hand blender or food processor whizz the soup until smooth. Stir in the crème fraîche and season with salt and pepper. Serve and enjoy.

Broccoli & Cheddar Soup

Ingredients

SERVES 4

309 calories per serving

175g (6oz) Cheddar cheese, grated (shredded)

1 head of broccoli, chopped

1 leek, chopped

1 courgette (zucchini), chopped

1 litre (1½ pints) chicken stock (broth)

150mls (5fl oz) single cream

Sea salt

Freshly ground black pepper

Method

Place the broccoli, leek and courgette (zucchini) in a saucepan and pour in the stock (broth). Bring them to the boil, reduce the heat and simmer for 15 minutes or until the vegetables are tender. Stir in the cream then using a hand blender or food processor blend until the soup becomes smooth. Add a little hot water or stock (broth) if you want to adjust the consistency. Season with salt and pepper and sprinkle with cheese.

Courgette (Zucchini) Fritters

Ingredients

450g (1lb) courgettes (zucchinis), grated (shredded)

100g (3½ oz) Parmesan cheese

3 cloves of garlic

3 spring onions (scallions)

2 eggs

1 teaspoon dried mixed herbs

1 tablespoon olive oil

Sprinkling of salt

SERVES 4

204 calories per serving

Method

Place the grated (shredded) courgette (zucchini) into a colander and sprinkle with a little salt. Allow it to sit for 30 minutes then squeeze out any excess moisture. Place the eggs, Parmesan, spring onions (scallions), garlic and dried herbs into a bowl and mix well with the courgettes. Scoop out a spoonful of the mixture and shape it into patties. Heat the oil in a frying pan, add the patties and cook for 2 minutes, turn them over and cook for another 2 minutes. Serve warm.

42

Taco Lettuce Wraps

Ingredients

450g (1lb) minced beef (ground beef)

100g (3½ oz) Cheddar cheese, grated

2 tomatoes, sliced

2 tablespoons tomato purée (paste)

1 romaine or iceberg lettuce, leaves washed and separated

½ teaspoon dried cumin

½ teaspoon paprika

½ teaspoon dried oregano

1 tablespoon olive oil

SERVES 4

386 calories per serving

Method

Heat the olive oil in a frying pan, add the meat, cumin, paprika and oregano and cook for 10 minutes. Add in the tomato purée (paste) and cook for another 5 minutes until the meat is completely cooked. Lay out the lettuce leaves and spoon some meat into each one. Add the tomato slices and sprinkle with cheese. Serve and eat immediately. Your choice of toppings can be varied to include sour cream, guacamole, mushrooms, onions, chillies or red peppers.

Mozzarella Slices

Ingredients

300g (11oz) mozzarella cheese, grated (shredded)

4 eggs

3 cloves of garlic, crushed

2 teaspoons dried oregano

1 cauliflower (approx.700g), grated (shredded)

Sea salt

Freshly ground black pepper

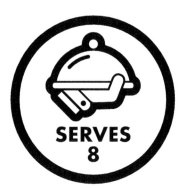

SERVES 8

157
calories
per serving

Method

Steam the cauliflower for 5 minutes or until tender and allow it to cool. Place the cauliflower in a bowl and combine it with the eggs, oregano, garlic and two thirds of the cheese. Season with salt and pepper. Grease 2 baking sheets. Divide the mixture in half and place it on the baking sheet and press it into a flat rectangular shape. Transfer the baking sheets to the oven and bake at 220C/440F for 20-25 minutes or until slightly golden. Remove them from the oven and sprinkle them with the remaining mozzarella cheese. Return them to the oven for 4-5 minutes or until the cheese has melted. Cut into slices and serve.

Piri Piri & Prawn Salad

Ingredients

8 king prawns (shrimps)
1 large handful of mixed lettuce leaves
1 small handful of fresh coriander (cilantro) leaves
1 tomato, chopped
½ avocado, stone removed, peeled and chopped
1 clove of garlic
1 small red chilli pepper, deseeded
½ red pepper (bell pepper), roughly chopped
1 tablespoons red wine vinegar
1 tablespoons olive oil

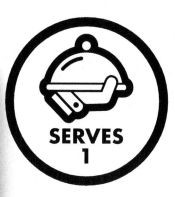

SERVES 1

344 calories per serving

Method

Place the red pepper (bell pepper), garlic, vinegar, oil and chilli into a blender and blitz until smooth. Transfer the mixture to a bowl and add the prawns. Allow them to marinate for at least 30 minutes. Heat a frying pan on high, add the prawns (shrimps) and cook them for around 5 minutes, or until they are pink and cooked through. Scatter the lettuce leaves on a plate and add the coriander (cilantro) tomato and avocado. Spoon the prawns and the sauce over the top. Eat straight away.

Creamy Garlic Mushroom Wraps

Ingredients

200g (7oz) mushroom, chopped

4 Romaine lettuce leaves

2 cloves of garlic, chopped

1 tablespoon crème fraîche

1 teaspoon olive oil

½ teaspoon mustard

1 teaspoon soy sauce

Sea salt

Freshly ground black pepper

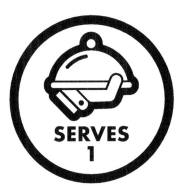

**SERVES
1**

98
calories
per serving

Method

Heat the oil in a frying pan, add the mushrooms, garlic, mustard and soy sauce and cook for around 5 minutes or until the mushrooms have softened. Stir in the crème fraîche and warm it thoroughly. Season with salt and pepper. Spoon some of the mixture into each of the lettuce leaves and eat straight away.

Prawn, Crab & Avocado Wraps

Ingredients

- 75g (3oz) peeled cooked prawns (shrimps)
- 75g (3oz) cooked crabmeat
- 2 spring onions (scallions) chopped
- 1 tomato, chopped
- 1 little gem lettuce
- 1/2 avocado, de-stoned, peeled and diced
- 2 teaspoons mayonnaise
- Squeeze of lemon juice
- Small handful of chives, chopped
- Wedge of lemon
- Sea salt
- Freshly ground black pepper

SERVES 1

391 calories per serving

Method

Place the mayonnaise and lemon juice in a bowl and mix well. Season with salt and pepper. Add the prawns, crabmeat, spring onions (scallions) and tomato into the mixture and stir. Separate the lettuce leaves and lay them onto a plate. Scatter some of the diced avocado into each lettuce leaf. Spoon some of the prawn mixture into each lettuce leaf. Sprinkle some chopped chives into each lettuce leaf. Chill before serving.

Szechuan Chicken Salad

Ingredients

450g (1lb) chicken, cut into strips (or turkey)
4 spring onions (scallions), chopped
2 tablespoons fresh coriander (cilantro) leaves, chopped
2 tomatoes, chopped
1 romaine lettuce, chopped
1 cucumber, deseeded and chopped
1 teaspoon ground Szechuan pepper
2 tablespoons sesame oil
Juice of 1 lime
1 tablespoon olive oil

SERVES 4

294 calories per serving

Method

Heat the olive oil in a pan, add the chicken strips and cook for 8 minutes or until the chicken is completely cooked. Remove it and let it cool. Place the chicken, cucumber, tomatoes and coriander (cilantro) in a bowl and stir in the sesame oil, Szechuan pepper, lime juice and spring onions (scallions). Scatter the lettuce on plates and scoop the chicken salad on top.

Herby Feta Aubergine Rolls

Ingredients

125g (4oz) feta cheese

2 tomatoes, chopped

6 asparagus spears

1 aubergine (eggplant) cut into 6 lengthways slices

1 tablespoon fresh basil, chopped

1 tablespoon fresh chives, chopped

2 tablespoons olive oil

SERVES 2

334
calories
per serving

Method

Heat the olive oil in a frying pan, add in the aubergine (eggplant) slices and cook for 2-3 minutes on each side. In the meantime, steam the asparagus for 5 minutes until it has softened. Place the aubergine slices onto plates and sprinkle some cheese, tomatoes and herbs onto each slice. Roll the aubergine slices up and secure it with a cocktail stick. Serve and enjoy.

Garlic Dough Balls

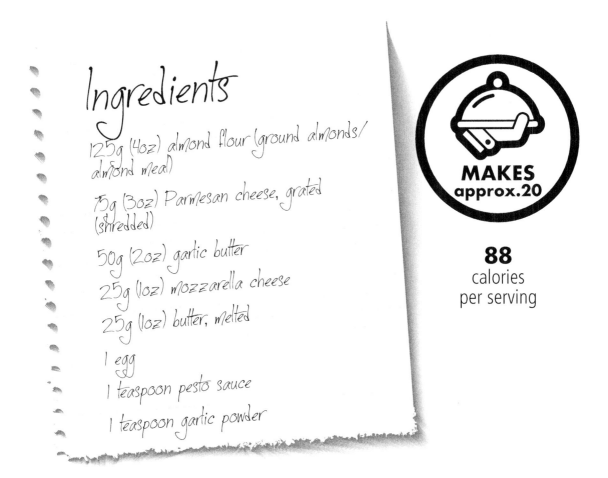

Ingredients

125g (4oz) almond flour (ground almonds/almond meal)

75g (3oz) Parmesan cheese, grated (shredded)

50g (2oz) garlic butter

25g (1oz) mozzarella cheese

25g (1oz) butter, melted

1 egg

1 teaspoon pesto sauce

1 teaspoon garlic powder

MAKES approx.20

88
calories
per serving

Method

Place all of the ingredients, apart from the garlic butter, into a bowl and mix them well. Grease and line a baking tray. Scoop out a tablespoon of the mixture and roll it into a ball. Repeat it for the remaining mixture. Transfer it to the oven and bake at 180C/360F for around 20 minutes, or until golden. Spread some garlic butter onto each dough ball. Enjoy them while they are still warm.

Prawn & Cannellini Avocados

Ingredients

300g (11oz) tinned cannellini beans, drained
300g (11oz) cooked, shelled prawns
2 avocados, halved with stone removed
1 red pepper (bell pepper), finely chopped
2 cloves of garlic, crushed
1 tablespoon fresh coriander (cilantro)
½ teaspoon ground paprika
2 tablespoons extra virgin olive oil
Juice of ½ lemon
Sea salt
Freshly ground black pepper

**SERVES
4**

333
calories
per serving

Method

Pour the lemon juice and olive oil into a bowl and mix well. Stir in the cannellini beans, prawns, red pepper (bell pepper), coriander (cilantro), garlic, paprika, salt and black pepper. Mix together until the ingredients are coated with the dressing. Serve the avocado halves onto plates and scoop the prawn mixture on top.

Bacon & Butterbean Salad

Ingredients

400g (14oz) tin butterbeans, drained

6 strips of bacon, chopped

3 tablespoons red wine vinegar

2 tablespoons fresh chives, chopped

2 tablespoons olive oil

1 teaspoon mustard

Sea salt

Freshly ground black pepper

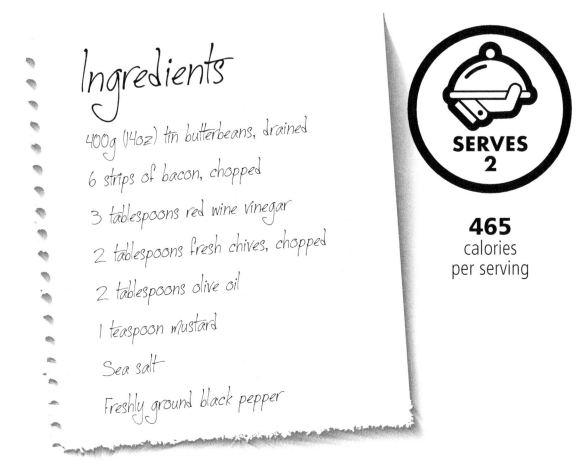

SERVES 2

465
calories
per serving

Method

Heat a frying pan, add the bacon and cook until crispy. Remove it and set it aside to cool. In a bowl, mix together the oil, vinegar, chives and mustard. Stir in the butterbeans and bacon. Season with salt and pepper. Chill before serving.

Italian Lentil Salad

Ingredients

450g (1lb) green lentils
100g (3½ oz) hazelnuts, chopped
2 spring onions (scallions), chopped
1 cucumber, peeled and diced
1 red pepper (bell pepper), sliced
1 handful of fresh basil
Zest and juice of 1 lemon
100mls (3½ fl oz) extra virgin olive oil
Sea salt
Freshly ground black pepper

SERVES 4

362
calories
per serving

Method

Cook the lentils according to the instructions then allow them to cool. Pour the olive oil and lemon juice into a jug and combine them. Season with salt and pepper. Place all the ingredients for the salad into a bowl and pour on the olive oil and lemon juice.

Lemon Lentil Salad

Ingredients

200g (7oz) Puy lentils
4 eggs
4 tomatoes, deseeded and chopped
4 spring onions (scallions), finely chopped
2 tablespoons olive oil
2 tablespoons parsley
2 large handfuls of washed spinach leaves
1 clove of garlic
Juice and rind of 1 lemon
Sea salt
Freshly ground black pepper

SERVES 4

231 calories per serving

Method

Place the lentils in a saucepan, cover them with water and bring them to the boil. Reduce the heat and cook for 20-25 minutes. Drain them once they are soft. Heat the olive oil in a saucepan, add the garlic and spring onions (scallions) and cook for 2 minutes. Stir in the tomatoes, lemon juice and rind. Cook for 2 minutes. Stir in the lentils and keep warm. In a pan of gently simmering water, poach the eggs until they are set but soft in the middle which should be 3-4 minutes. Scatter the spinach leaves onto plates, serve the lentils and top off with a poached egg. Season with salt and pepper.

Halloumi & Asparagus Salad

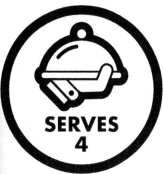

SERVES 4

257 calories per serving

Ingredients

450g (1lb) asparagus

250g (9oz) halloumi cheese, cut into slices

2 large handfuls of spinach leaves

1 tablespoon olive oil

Sea salt

Freshly ground black pepper

Method

Heat the olive oil in a frying pan and cook the asparagus for 4 minutes or until tender. Remove, set aside and keep warm. Place the halloumi in the frying pan and cook for 2 minutes on each side until golden. Serve the spinach leaves onto plates and add the asparagus and halloumi slices. Season with salt and pepper.

Spiced Chicken & Courgette Salad

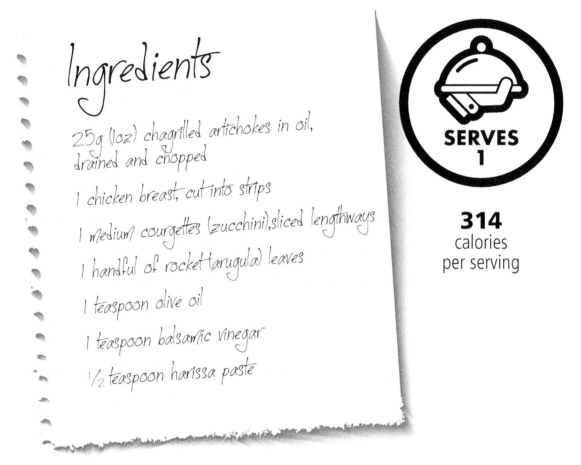

Ingredients

25g (1oz) chagrilled artichokes in oil, drained and chopped

1 chicken breast, cut into strips

1 medium courgettes (zucchini), sliced lengthways

1 handful of rocket (arugula) leaves

1 teaspoon olive oil

1 teaspoon balsamic vinegar

½ teaspoon harissa paste

SERVES 1

314 calories per serving

Method

Place the harissa paste and olive oil in a bowl and coat the chicken in the mixture. Heat a griddle pan on a high heat and lay the courgette (zucchini) slices on it. Cook them until they have softened slightly then set them aside and keep warm. Place the chicken in the pan and cook it for around 6 minutes or until cooked completely, turning it over halfway through. Scatter the rocket (arugula) leaves onto a plate together with the artichoke pieces. Add the courgette and chicken to the salad. Drizzle the balsamic vinegar over the top. Serve and eat straight away.

Avocado Baked Eggs

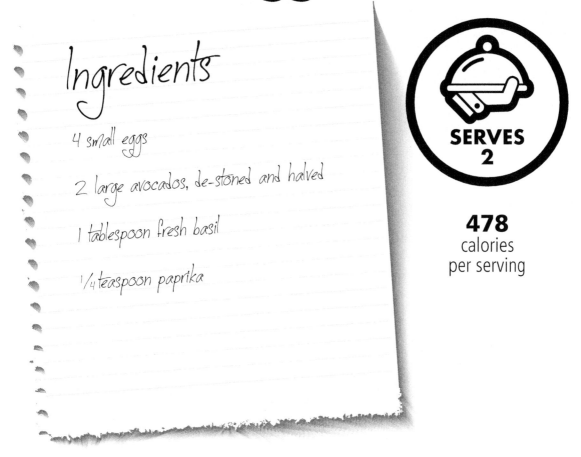

Ingredients

4 small eggs

2 large avocados, de-stoned and halved

1 tablespoon fresh basil

1/4 teaspoon paprika

SERVES 2

478 calories per serving

Method

Depending on the size you may need to scoop out a little avocado flesh to make room for the egg. Crack the egg into the avocado. Sprinkle with paprika. Place them in an oven-proof dish. Transfer them to the oven and bake at 220C/440F for 18-20 minutes. Sprinkle with basil and serve.

MAIN MEALS

Steak & Chorizo Kebabs

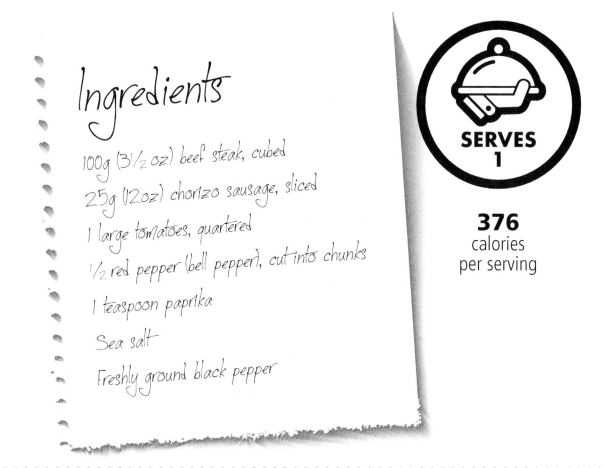

Ingredients

100g (3½ oz) beef steak, cubed

25g (12oz) chorizo sausage, sliced

1 large tomatoes, quartered

½ red pepper (bell pepper), cut into chunks

1 teaspoon paprika

Sea salt

Freshly ground black pepper

**SERVES
1**

376
calories
per serving

Method

Sprinkle the steak with the paprika and season with salt and pepper. Thread the steak, tomato, pepper and chorizo alternately onto skewers. Place them under a hot grill (broiler) for around 10 minutes or until the steak is cooked, turning during cooking to ensure even cooking.

Low-Carb Turkey Lasagne

Ingredients

450g (1lb) minced (ground) turkey

400g (14oz) ricotta cheese

300g (11oz) mozzarella cheese, grated (shredded)

2 x 400g (14oz) tin of chopped tomatoes

25g (1oz) Parmesan cheese

4 courgettes (zucchinis) sliced lengthways

3 tablespoons fresh basil, chopped

2 cloves of garlic, crushed

1 onion, chopped

1 red pepper (bell pepper), chopped

1 teaspoon dried oregano

1 egg

1 tablespoon olive oil

Sea salt

SERVES 6

443 calories per serving

Method

Grease a baking sheet and lay the courgette (zucchini) slices on it. Season with salt, transfer it to the oven and bake at 190C/375F for 15 minutes. In the meantime, heat the oil in a saucepan, add the onions, garlic and red pepper (bell pepper) and cook for 5 minutes. Add in the turkey and cook for 4 minutes. Stir in the tomatoes, basil and oregano. Bring it to the boil, reduce the heat and simmer for 30 minutes. In a bowl combine the egg and ricotta cheese then set aside. When the turkey mixture is cooked, spoon half of it into an ovenproof dish. Add a layer of the baked courgettes then spoon on half of the ricotta mixture and a layer of mozzarella, repeat with the remaining mixture. Sprinkle Parmesan on top. Transfer it to the oven and bake at 375F/180C for 40 minutes. Serve with a leafy green salad.

Lemon & Herb Lamb Chops

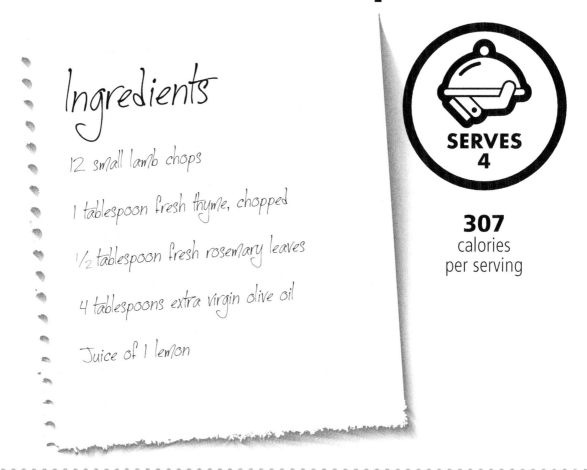

Ingredients

12 small lamb chops

1 tablespoon fresh thyme, chopped

1/2 tablespoon fresh rosemary leaves

4 tablespoons extra virgin olive oil

Juice of 1 lemon

SERVES 4

307 calories per serving

Method

Pour the oil into a bowl and stir in the lemon juice, rosemary and thyme. Place the lamb chops in the mixture and allow it to marinate for at least 1 hour or overnight if you can. Transfer the chops to a hot grill (broiler) and cook for 5 minutes on either side or until the chops are cooked to your liking. Serve with courgette 'spaghetti' and a salad.

Thai Chicken Curry

SERVES 1

362
calories
per serving

Ingredients

3 spring onions (scallions), chopped

50g (2oz) broccoli, broken into small florets

1 chicken breast, chopped

1 teaspoon coconut oil

1/2 red pepper (bell pepper), chopped

2 teaspoons Thai red curry paste

Small bunch of coriander leaves (cilantro), chopped

100mls (3½ fl oz) coconut milk

Method

Heat the coconut oil in a large pan. Add the chicken and cook it for 4 minutes, stirring occassionally. Add the spring onions (scallions), pepper and broccoli and cook for 2 minutes. Add the curry paste and coconut milk and simmer for 15 minutes. Add the chopped coriander (cilantro) and stir. Serve on it's own or with a heap of vegetables.

Bean & Quinoa Casserole

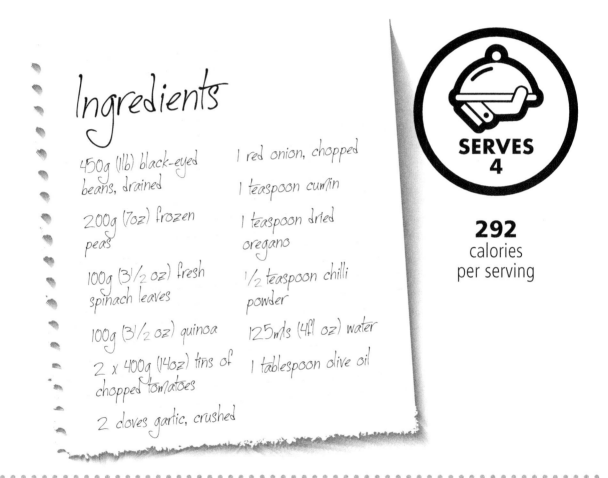

Ingredients

450g (1lb) black-eyed beans, drained

200g (7oz) frozen peas

100g (3½ oz) fresh spinach leaves

100g (3½ oz) quinoa

2 x 400g (14oz) tins of chopped tomatoes

2 cloves garlic, crushed

1 red onion, chopped

1 teaspoon cumin

1 teaspoon dried oregano

½ teaspoon chilli powder

125mls (4fl oz) water

1 tablespoon olive oil

**SERVES
4**

292
calories
per serving

Method

Heat the oil in a saucepan, add the onion and garlic and cook for 5 minutes. Transfer to an ovenproof dish. Add in the quinoa, tomatoes, cumin, oregano and chilli powder. Place the dish in the oven and cook at 180C/360F for 20 minutes. Stir in the beans, peas and water. Cover with foil and cook for 20 minutes. Remove it from the oven, stir in the spinach and allow it to wilt for a couple of minutes before serving.

Chicken & Prawn Stir-Fry

Ingredients

50g (2oz) mushrooms, sliced

25g (1oz) bamboo shoots

25g (1oz) water chestnuts, drained

6 king prawns (shrimps), shelled

1 chicken breast, chopped

1/2 red pepper (bell pepper), sliced

1/2 courgette (zucchini) sliced

2 spring onions (scallions), chopped

2 teaspoons olive oil

1 teaspoon lemon juice

1 teaspoon soy sauce

1/2 teaspoon ground ginger

1 clove of garlic, chopped

Sea salt

Freshly ground black pepper

**SERVES
1**

335
calories
per serving

Method

Place the lemon juice, ginger, garlic and soy sauce in a bowl and mix well. Add in the chicken and coat it in the mixture. Cover and allow it to marinate for at least 30 minutes. Heat the oil in a frying pan. Add the chicken and cook it for 3-4 minutes then remove it and set aside. Add the prawns (shrimps), red pepper (bell pepper), courgette (zucchini), spring onions (scallions), mushrooms, bamboo shoots and water chestnuts and cook for 3 minutes. Return the chicken to the frying pan and continue cooking until it is completely done. Season with salt and pepper and serve.

Salmon, Butter Beans & Yogurt Dressing

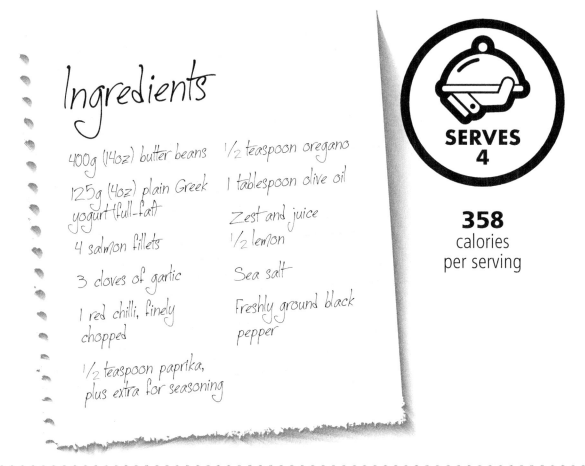

Ingredients

400g (14oz) butter beans

125g (4oz) plain Greek yogurt (full-fat)

4 salmon fillets

3 cloves of garlic

1 red chilli, finely chopped

1/2 teaspoon paprika, plus extra for seasoning

1/2 teaspoon oregano

1 tablespoon olive oil

Zest and juice 1/2 lemon

Sea salt

Freshly ground black pepper

SERVES 4

358 calories per serving

Method

Place the yogurt into a bowl and add in the lemon juice and paprika. Heat the oil in a pan, add the oregano, garlic and chilli and warm them for 2 minutes. Add in the butter beans and lemon zest and warm them through. Sprinkle the paprika over the salmon and season it with salt and pepper. Place the salmon fillets under a hot grill (broiler) and cook for around 8 minutes, or until completely cooked, turning half way through. Serve the salmon with the butter beans and a dollop of yogurt dressing.

Hunter's Chicken

Ingredients

400g (14oz) broccoli florets

125g (4oz) cheese, grated (shredded)

8 slices of bacon

4 chicken breasts

1 onion, chopped

250g (8oz) tomato passata (sauce)

3 tablespoons balsamic vinegar

1 tablespoon olive oil

**SERVES
4**

476
calories
per serving

Method

Heat the oil in a frying pan, add the onion and cook for 5 minutes. Add the passata and balsamic and cook for 10 minutes to reduce the mixture. Place the chicken flat-side down on a lightly greased ovenproof and make an incision to make room for the sauce. Spoon the sauce into the incision. Wrap two slices of bacon around each chicken breast. Transfer the chicken to the oven and cook for 25 minutes. Scatter the cheese over the chicken breasts and return them to the oven for 5 minutes or until the cheese is bubbling. In the meantime steam or boil the broccoli for 5 minutes. Serve the broccoli onto plates and add the chicken.

Tomato & Pesto Chicken

SERVES 1

363
calories
per serving

Ingredients

200g (7oz) tinned chopped tomatoes

25g (1oz) sundried tomatoes, chopped

2 teaspoons pesto

1 teaspoon pine nuts

1 chicken breast

1 small handful of fresh basil, chopped

1 large handful of fresh mixed lettuce leaves

Method

Place the tinned tomatoes in an ovenproof dish and add in the sundried tomatoes and basil and stir well. Coat both sides of the chicken breast with the pesto then lay it on top of the tomatoes. Cook in the oven at 200C/400F for around 30 minutes or until the chicken is completely cooked. Scatter the salad leaves onto a plate. Serve the chicken on top with a scattering of pine nuts.

Tandoori Chicken Salad

Ingredients

50g (2oz) plain (unflavoured) yogurt
4cm (2 inch) chunk of cucumber, diced
1 chicken breast
1 clove of garlic, crushed
1 teaspoon tandoori spice mix
1 handful of mixed lettuce leaves
1 ripe tomato, chopped
1 tablespoon fresh coriander (cilantro), chopped
½ red pepper (bell pepper), chopped

**SERVES
1**

260
calories
per serving

Method

Place the yogurt in a bowl and stir in the spice mix and garlic. Coat the chicken in the marinade and chill in the fridge for one hour (or longer if you can) to allow it to marinate. When you are ready to cook it, lay the chicken in an ovenproof dish. Cook at 180C/360F for 20 minutes, or until the chicken is completely cooked. Remove it from the oven and allow it to cool. Scatter the lettuce, cucumber, tomato and pepper onto a plate. Slice the chicken and lay it on top of the salad. Sprinkle the coriander (cilantro) on top.

Vegetarian Chilli

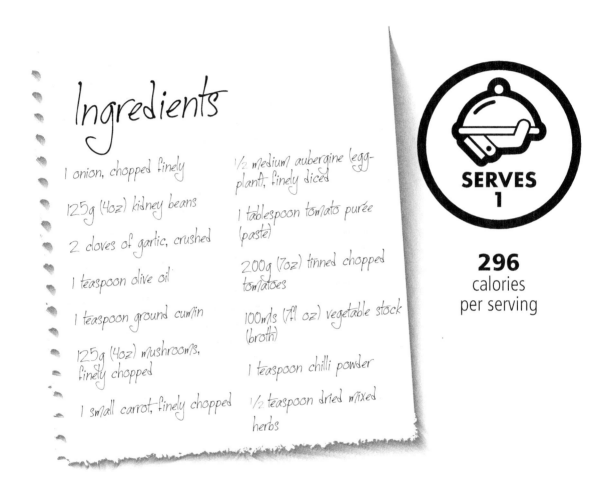

Ingredients

1 onion, chopped finely

125g (4oz) kidney beans

2 cloves of garlic, crushed

1 teaspoon olive oil

1 teaspoon ground cumin

125g (4oz) mushrooms, finely chopped

1 small carrot, finely chopped

½ medium aubergine (eggplant), finely diced

1 tablespoon tomato purée (paste)

200g (7oz) tinned chopped tomatoes

100mls (7fl oz) vegetable stock (broth)

1 teaspoon chilli powder

½ teaspoon dried mixed herbs

SERVES 1

296 calories per serving

Method

In a large saucepan, heat the olive oil. Add the onion and garlic and soften slightly. Add the mushrooms, carrot, tinned tomatoes, aubergine (eggplant), tomato purée (paste), vegetable stock (broth), chilli, cumin and mixed herbs. Bring to the boil then simmer for 30 minutes, stirring occasionally. Add the kidney beans and cook for another 10 minutes. You can serve it into romaine or iceberg lettuce leaves and add some cheese and/or guacamole.

Tuna Casserole

Ingredients

4 tuna steaks

2 red onions, chopped

2 stalks of celery

2 x 400g (2 x 14oz) tins of chopped tomatoes

2 cloves of garlic

1 tablespoon olive oil

1 lemon, thinly sliced

1 tablespoon tomato purée (paste)

2 tablespoons fresh oregano, chopped

Sea salt

Freshly ground black pepper

**SERVES
4**

229
calories
per serving

Method

Heat the oil in a saucepan and add the celery, garlic and onions and fry for 5 minutes until the vegetables have softened. Add in the tinned tomatoes, oregano, tomato puree (paste) and lemon slices. Bring to the boil and simmer, stirring, for 5 minutes. Season with salt and pepper. Place the fish in the tomato mixture. Simmer gently for 12-14 minutes until the fish is cooked. Serve the fish onto plates and pour the sauce on top. Garnish with a little oregano.

Tomato & Herb Stuffed Chicken

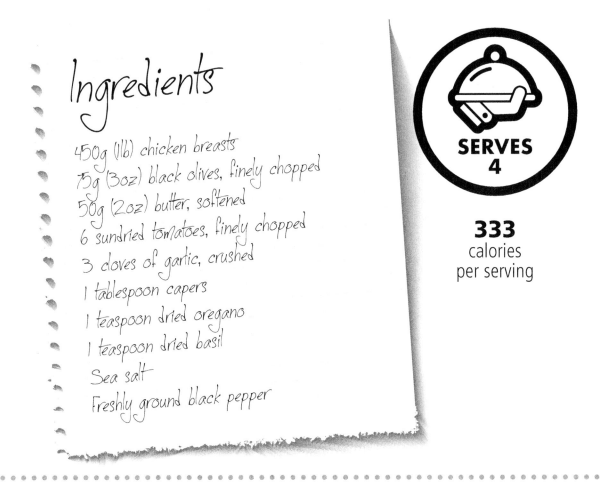

Ingredients

450g (1lb) chicken breasts
75g (3oz) black olives, finely chopped
50g (2oz) butter, softened
6 sundried tomatoes, finely chopped
3 cloves of garlic, crushed
1 tablespoon capers
1 teaspoon dried oregano
1 teaspoon dried basil
Sea salt
Freshly ground black pepper

SERVES 4

333
calories
per serving

Method

Place the olives, tomatoes, garlic, dried herbs and capers into a bowl and stir. Add in the softened butter and capers and mix well. Make an incision in each chicken breast to make a pocket for the butter mixture. Spoon the mixture inside each of the chicken breasts. Season with salt and pepper and wrap each one in tin foil. Transfer them to the oven and cook at 190C/375F for 25 minutes.

Lemon & Coriander (Cilantro) Chicken

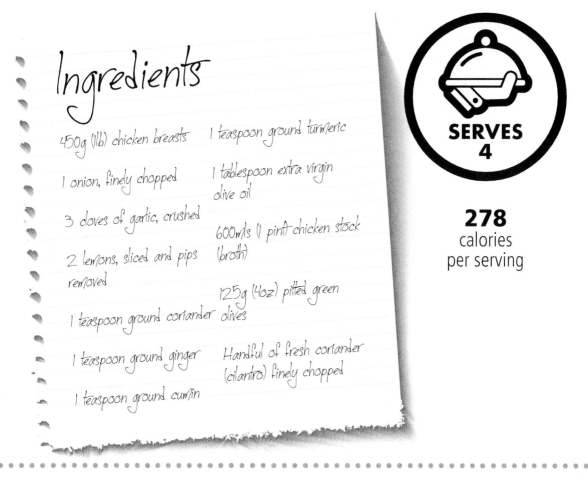

Ingredients

450g (1lb) chicken breasts

1 onion, finely chopped

3 cloves of garlic, crushed

2 lemons, sliced and pips removed

1 teaspoon ground coriander

1 teaspoon ground ginger

1 teaspoon ground cumin

1 teaspoon ground turmeric

1 tablespoon extra virgin olive oil

600mls (1 pint) chicken stock (broth)

125g (4oz) pitted green olives

Handful of fresh coriander (cilantro) finely chopped

SERVES 4

278 calories per serving

Method

Heat the oil in a saucepan, add the onion and cook for 5 minutes until softened. Add the garlic, cumin, turmeric, ginger and ground coriander (cilantro) and cook for 1 minute. Add the chicken and brown it. Add the slices of lemon and chicken stock (broth). Bring it to the boil, reduce the heat and simmer for 30 minutes. Stir in the fresh coriander (cilantro) and olives. Warm the olives through and then serve.

Cheesy Quinoa Cakes

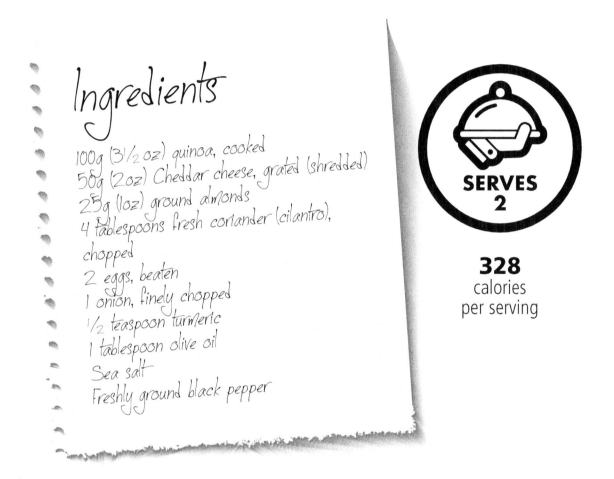

Ingredients

100g (3½ oz) quinoa, cooked
50g (2oz) Cheddar cheese, grated (shredded)
25g (1oz) ground almonds
4 tablespoons fresh coriander (cilantro), chopped
2 eggs, beaten
1 onion, finely chopped
½ teaspoon turmeric
1 tablespoon olive oil
Sea salt
Freshly ground black pepper

SERVES 2

328 calories per serving

Method

In a bowl, combine the eggs, onion, coriander (cilantro), turmeric, cheese, almonds and season with salt and pepper. Stir in the quinoa and mix well. With clean hands, form 8 small patties. Heat the olive oil in a frying pan and add the quinoa cakes. Cook for 3-4 minutes on either side until slightly golden.

Salmon Kebabs

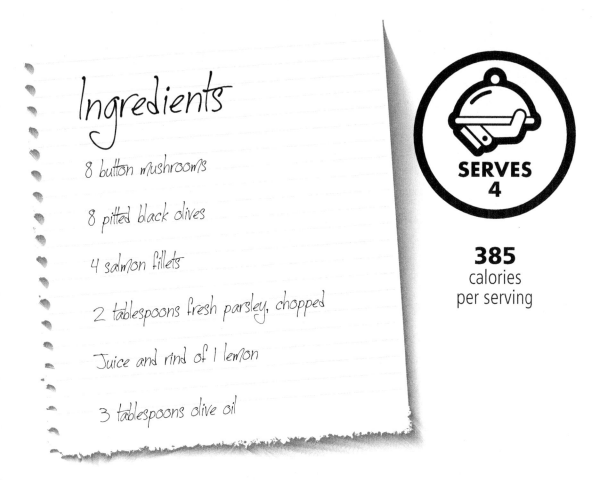

Ingredients

8 button mushrooms

8 pitted black olives

4 salmon fillets

2 tablespoons fresh parsley, chopped

Juice and rind of 1 lemon

3 tablespoons olive oil

SERVES 4

385 calories per serving

Method

Cut the salmon into chunks and place them in a bowl. Squeeze in the lemon juice and add the rind, olive oil and parsley and coat the salmon in the mixture. Add the mushrooms and coat them in the dressing too. Thread the fish, olives and mushrooms onto skewers. Place them under a hot grill (broiler) and cook for 4-5 minutes turning occasionally. Serve the kebabs and drizzle them with the remaining dressing.

Coconut & Vegetable Curry

Ingredients

200g (7oz) tofu, cubed

200g (7oz) mushrooms, chopped

125g (4oz) green beans, chopped

2 tablespoons fresh coriander (cilantro), chopped

1 tablespoon medium curry powder

1 teaspoon cumin

1 teaspoon turmeric

1 teaspoon ground ginger

400mls (14fl oz) full-fat coconut milk

Sea salt

Freshly ground black pepper

SERVES 4

204 calories per serving

Method

Warm the coconut milk in a saucepan then add in the curry powder, cumin, ginger and turmeric and mix it well. Add the mushrooms, green beans, tofu and stir. Bring it to the boil, reduce the heat and simmer for 8-10 minutes until the vegetables are soft. Sprinkle with coriander (cilantro) and serve with cauliflower rice.

Spinach & Cheese Stuffed Chicken

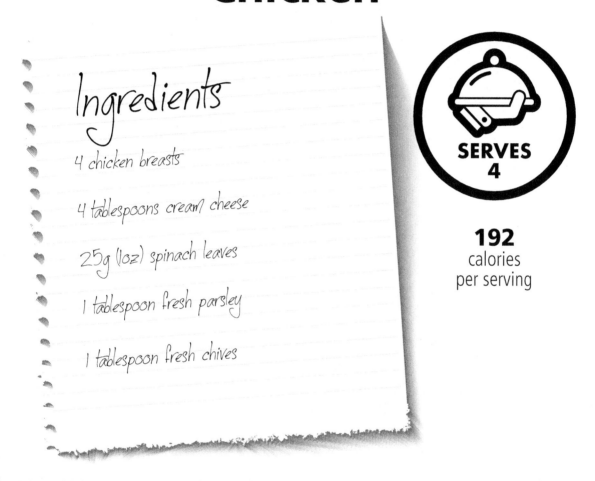

Ingredients

4 chicken breasts

4 tablespoons cream cheese

25g (1oz) spinach leaves

1 tablespoon fresh parsley

1 tablespoon fresh chives

SERVES 4

192 calories per serving

Method

In a bowl, combine the cream cheese, spinach and herbs until it's well mixed. Carefully make an incision on the underside of the chicken breast, wide enough to contain some cheese mixture. Spoon some of the mixture into the incision and press the chicken back together. Repeat for the remaining mixture. Place the stuffed chicken in an ovenproof dish. Transfer to the oven and bake at 180C/360F for around 30 minutes or until the chicken is completely cooked. Serve with a large green leafy salad. Enjoy.

Marinated Spare Ribs

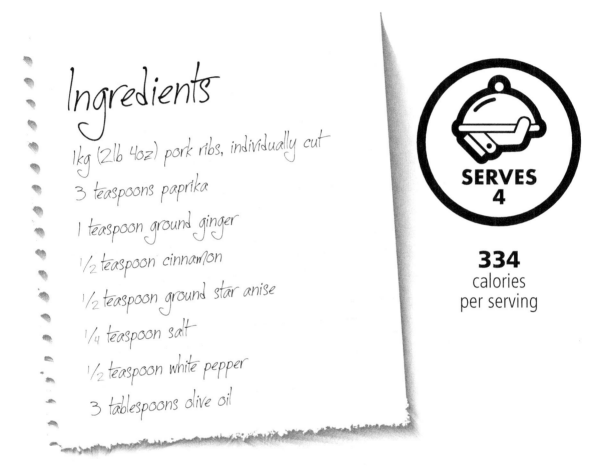

Ingredients

1kg (2lb 4oz) pork ribs, individually cut

3 teaspoons paprika

1 teaspoon ground ginger

1/2 teaspoon cinnamon

1/2 teaspoon ground star anise

1/4 teaspoon salt

1/2 teaspoon white pepper

3 tablespoons olive oil

SERVES 4

334 calories per serving

Method

Place the spices, salt, pepper and oil in a bowl and combine. Coat the ribs with the spice mixture and coat them thoroughly. Cover them and allow them to marinate for 30 minutes or overnight if you can. Place the pork ribs in a roasting tin, transfer them to the oven and cook at 180C/360F for 35-40 minutes. Serve onto a large plate for sharing.

Mini Cauliflower Pizza Bases

Ingredients

350g (12 oz) mozzarella cheese, grated (shredded)

2 eggs

1 head of cauliflower approx 700g (1½ lb), grated (shredded)

1 teaspoon dried oregano

1 teaspoon dried basil

1 teaspoon garlic powder

1 tomato, sliced

Handful of fresh basil leaves, chopped

200g (7oz) passata/ tomato sauce

SERVES 6

219 calories per serving

Method

Steam the grated (shredded) cauliflower for 5 minutes then allow it to cool. Place the cooked cauliflower in a bowl and add the eggs, half the cheese, all of the dried herbs and garlic and mix everything together really well. Grease two baking sheets. Divide the mixture into 12 and roll it into balls. Place them on a baking sheet and press them down until flat and round mini pizza bases. Transfer them to the oven and bake at 220C/440F for 12 minutes until lightly golden. Top each pizza base with a little passata, the remaining mozzarella and tomato and basil. Place the pizzas under a grill (broiler) and cook for 4-5 minutes or until the cheese has melted. Enjoy.

Parmesan Chicken

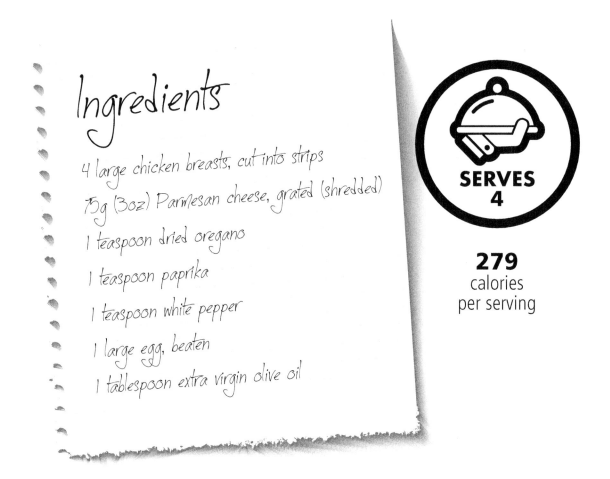

Ingredients

4 large chicken breasts, cut into strips

75g (3oz) Parmesan cheese, grated (shredded)

1 teaspoon dried oregano

1 teaspoon paprika

1 teaspoon white pepper

1 large egg, beaten

1 tablespoon extra virgin olive oil

SERVES 4

279 calories per serving

Method

On a plate, combine the Parmesan cheese with the oregano, paprika and pepper. Dip the chicken strips in the beaten egg and then coat them liberally with the Parmesan mixture. Heat the olive oil in a frying pan, add the chicken strips and cook them for around 4 or 5 minutes on each side, or until they are completely cooked.

Salt & Pepper Chicken Strips

Ingredients

1 large chicken breast (approx. 150g (5oz), cut into strips

3 spring onions (scallions), finely chopped

1 clove of garlic, crushed

1/2 teaspoon sea salt

1/2 teaspoon Szechuan pepper

1/2 teaspoon freshly ground black pepper

1/2 teaspoon chilli powder

1 teaspoon olive oil

SERVES 1

284 calories per serving

Method

Place the salt, Szechuan pepper, chilli powder, garlic and black pepper into a bowl. Place the chicken in a bowl and coat it in the mixture. Heat the oil in a frying pan, add the chicken and cook for 8-10 minutes until completely cooked. Scatter in the spring onions (scallions) and cook for 1 minute. Serve on their own or with salad or vegetables.

Steak With Chilli & Coriander Salsa

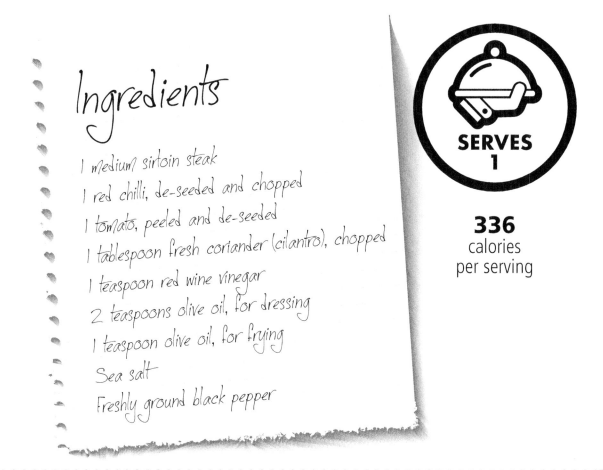

Ingredients

1 medium sirloin steak

1 red chilli, de-seeded and chopped

1 tomato, peeled and de-seeded

1 tablespoon fresh coriander (cilantro), chopped

1 teaspoon red wine vinegar

2 teaspoons olive oil, for dressing

1 teaspoon olive oil, for frying

Sea salt

Freshly ground black pepper

SERVES 1

336 calories per serving

Method

Place the tomato, chilli, coriander (cilantro), oil and vinegar into a bowl and mix well. Season with salt and pepper. Heat a teaspoon of olive oil in a frying pan. Place the steak in the pan and cook for 2-3 minutes if you like it rare, 4 minutes each side if you like it medium or 5-6 minutes on each side if you like it well done. Serve the steak and add the salsa to the side. Enjoy with salad.

Mediterranean Cod

Ingredients

4 cod fillets

1 onion, chopped

2 cloves of garlic, crushed

1 x 400g (14oz) tin of chopped tomatoes

75g (3oz) pitted black olives, sliced

2 tablespoons olive oil

100mls (3½ fl oz) vegetable or chicken stock (broth)

Handful of fresh parsley

SERVES 4

223
calories
per serving

Method

Heat the oil in a frying pan, add the onions and garlic and cook for 5 minutes. Add in chopped tomatoes, parsley, olives and stock. Bring it to the boil and simmer for 5 minutes. Add the cod fillets in the sauce and simmer gently for 5-6 minutes or until the fish is white and thoroughly cooked.

Rack of Lamb With Cucumber & Hummus

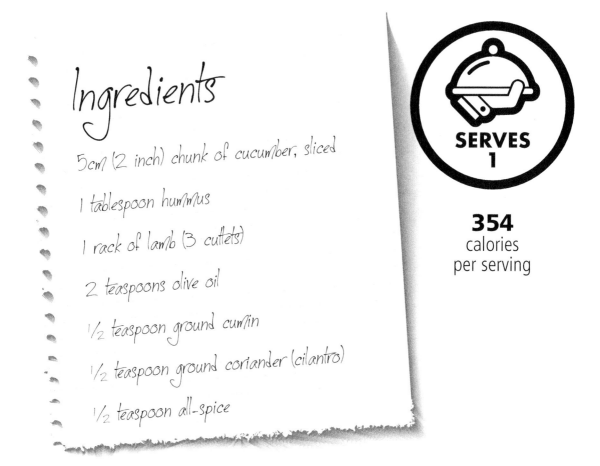

SERVES 1

354 calories per serving

Ingredients

5cm (2 inch) chunk of cucumber, sliced

1 tablespoon hummus

1 rack of lamb (3 cutlets)

2 teaspoons olive oil

1/2 teaspoon ground cumin

1/2 teaspoon ground coriander (cilantro)

1/2 teaspoon all-spice

Method

Place the oil, cumin, coriander (cilantro) and all-spice into a bowl and mix well. Coat the lamb in the mixture. Place the lamb in a roasting tin and cook in the oven at 220C/445F for 15-20 minutes or until the lamb has browned. Place the cucumber onto a plate and add a dollop of hummus and serve the lamb. Enjoy straight away.

Pork Steaks, Peppers & Beans

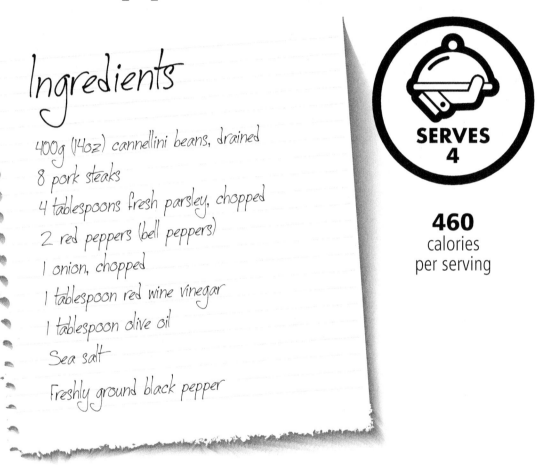

Ingredients

400g (14oz) cannellini beans, drained

8 pork steaks

4 tablespoons fresh parsley, chopped

2 red peppers (bell peppers)

1 onion, chopped

1 tablespoon red wine vinegar

1 tablespoon olive oil

Sea salt

Freshly ground black pepper

SERVES 4

460
calories
per serving

Method

Season the pork steaks with salt and pepper. Heat the olive oil in a frying pan, add the pork and cook for around 3 minutes on each side. Remove them, set aside and keep them warm. Add the peppers (bell peppers) and onion to the pan and cook for 5 minutes until the vegetables have softened. Add the parsley, vinegar and beans and warm them thoroughly. Serve the pork steaks and spoon the vegetables over the top. Enjoy.

Mediterranean Duck & Cannellini Beans

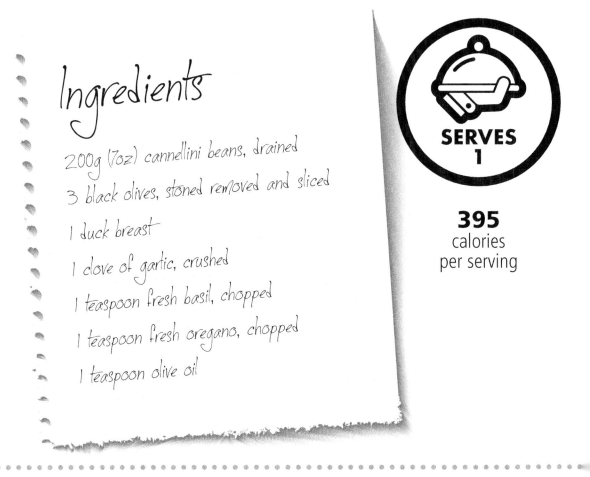

SERVES 1

395 calories per serving

Ingredients

200g (7oz) cannellini beans, drained

3 black olives, stoned removed and sliced

1 duck breast

1 clove of garlic, crushed

1 teaspoon fresh basil, chopped

1 teaspoon fresh oregano, chopped

1 teaspoon olive oil

Method

Lay the duck on a chopping board and make several incisions then push the garlic, basil and oregano into the duck. Place the duck breast under a hot grill (broiler) and cook on each side for 5 minutes or longer if you like it well done. In the meantime, heat the oil in a frying pan, add the beans and olives and cook for 4-5 minutes or until they have warmed through. Serve the beans onto a plate and place the duck on top. Serve and eat straight away.

Mozzarella Roast Vegetables

Ingredients

25g (1oz) mozzarella cheese, grated (shredded)

4 florets of broccoli, roughly chopped

1 small courgette (zucchini), chopped

1 red pepper (bell pepper), chopped

1 medium tomato, chopped

½ onion, peeled and roughly chopped

½ teaspoon mixed herbs

1 teaspoon olive oil

**SERVES
1**

209
calories
per serving

Method

Place all of the ingredients, apart from the mozzarella, into a large ovenproof dish and mix them well. Place the vegetables in the oven and cook them at 200C/400F for 20 minutes. Remove the dish from the oven and sprinkle over the mozzarella cheese. Return it to the oven and continue cooking for 5-10 minutes when the cheese is completely melted. Use as a side dish to go along with chicken, meat and fish meals instead of potatoes or pasta.

Fresh Basil, Mozzarella & Tomato Chicken

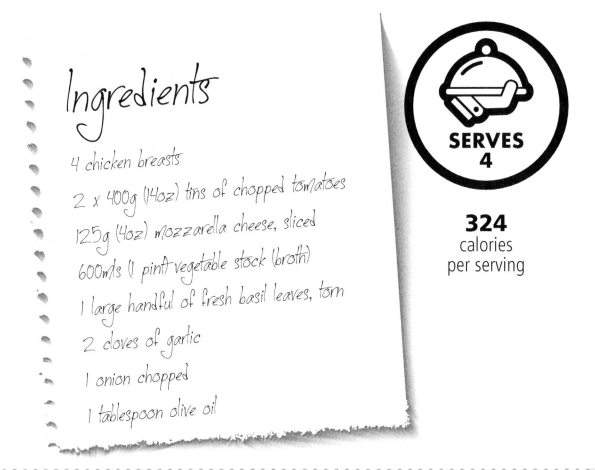

Ingredients

4 chicken breasts

2 x 400g (14oz) tins of chopped tomatoes

125g (4oz) mozzarella cheese, sliced

600mls (1 pint) vegetable stock (broth)

1 large handful of fresh basil leaves, torn

2 cloves of garlic

1 onion chopped

1 tablespoon olive oil

SERVES 4

324 calories per serving

Method

Heat the olive oil in a frying pan, add the onion and garlic and cook for 5 minutes or until softened. Add the chopped tomatoes and stock (broth). Add in the basil leaves, bring it to the boil, reduce the heat and simmer for 5 minutes. Place the chicken in an ovenproof dish. Cover the chicken with the sauce and add slices of mozzarella to the dish. Transfer it to the oven and cook at 190C/375F for around 20 minutes or until the chicken is completely cooked. Serve with a leafy green salad.

Beef Stir-Fry

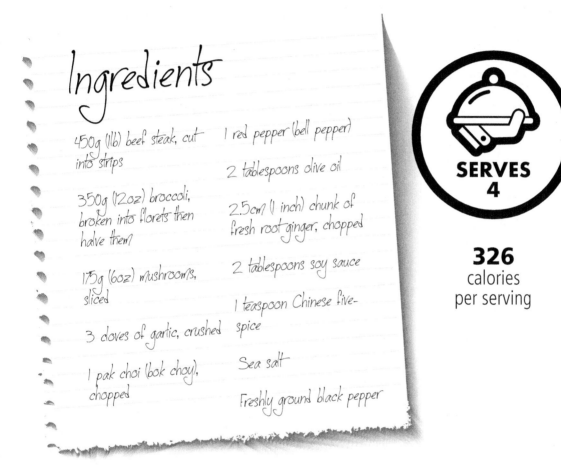

Ingredients

450g (1lb) beef steak, cut into strips

350g (12oz) broccoli, broken into florets then halve them

175g (6oz) mushrooms, sliced

3 cloves of garlic, crushed

1 pak choi (bok choy), chopped

1 red pepper (bell pepper)

2 tablespoons olive oil

2.5cm (1 inch) chunk of fresh root ginger, chopped

2 tablespoons soy sauce

1 teaspoon Chinese five-spice

Sea salt

Freshly ground black pepper

SERVES 4

326 calories per serving

Method

Heat a tablespoon of olive oil in a large frying pan or wok until it begins to smoke. Add the beef and brown it then remove and set aside. Heat the remaining olive oil and mushrooms, ginger, five-spice and garlic and cook for 3 minutes. Add in the broccoli and red pepper (bell pepper) and cook for 4 minutes. Stir in the pak choi (bok choy) and cook until softened. Add the beef strips and stir in the soy sauce. Season with salt and pepper. Serve and enjoy.

Mustard & Garlic Prawns

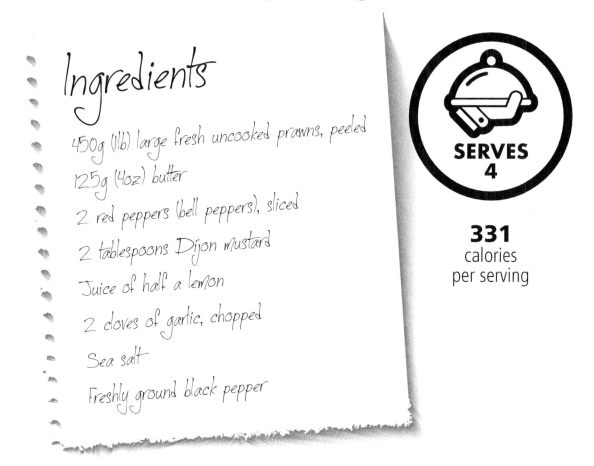

Ingredients

450g (1lb) large fresh uncooked prawns, peeled

125g (4oz) butter

2 red peppers (bell peppers), sliced

2 tablespoons Dijon mustard

Juice of half a lemon

2 cloves of garlic, chopped

Sea salt

Freshly ground black pepper

SERVES 4

331 calories per serving

Method

Place the prawns in an ovenproof dish and scatter the red peppers (bell peppers) into the dish. Heat the butter in a small saucepan and stir in the mustard, garlic and lemon juice. Warm the mixture until the butter has melted. Pour the butter over the prawns and peppers. Season with salt and pepper. Transfer to the oven and bake at 220C/425F for 15 minutes or until the prawns are pink and completely cooked.

Cottage Pie

Ingredients

450g (1lb) beef mince (ground beef)

400g (14oz) tinned chopped tomatoes

1 carrot, peeled and finely chopped

1 cauliflower (approx 700g (1 1/2 lb) broken into florets

1 leek, trimmed and finely chopped

1 onion, chopped

1 tablespoon soy sauce

1 tablespoon tomato purée (paste)

1 tablespoon olive oil

1 small handful fresh parsley, chopped

300mls (1/2 pint) beef stock (broth)

SERVES 4

370 calories per serving

Method

Heat the oil in a saucepan, add the mince and cook for 3 minutes. Add in the carrot and onion and cook for 5 minutes. Add in the tomatoes, tomato purée, soy sauce, parsley and stock (broth). Bring it to the boil, reduce the heat and simmer for 30 minutes. In the meantime, boil the cauliflower until tender then drain it. Mash until soft. Fry the leeks in a pan until they become soft. Combine the leeks with the mashed cauliflower. Transfer the meat to an ovenproof dish and spoon the cauliflower mixture on top. Place the dish in the oven at 200C/400F for around 30 minutes or golden on top.

Lamb Shank Casserole

SERVES 2

432 calories per serving

Ingredients

2 lamb shanks

4 large mushrooms, chopped

3 carrots, chopped

3 cloves of garlic, crushed

2 large tomatoes, chopped

1 onion, finely chopped

2 tablespoons tomato purée (paste)

2 large sprigs of rosemary

1 bouquet garni

½ bulb of fennel, chopped

750ml (1½ pints) beef vegetable stock (broth)

2 tablespoons olive oil

Method

Heat the oil in a large saucepan and add the lamb, turning occasionally until it is brown all over. Transfer the lamb to a bowl and set aside. Add the onion, fennel, mushrooms, carrots and garlic to the saucepan and cook for 5 minutes. Return the lamb to the saucepan and add in the stock, tomatoes, tomato purée (paste), rosemary, and bouquet garni. Transfer to an oven-proof dish, cover and cook in the oven at 200C/400F for 2 hours. Check half way through cooking and add extra stock (broth) or water if necessary. Remove the bouquet garni. Serve and enjoy.

Harissa Meatballs & Yogurt Dip

Ingredients

450g (1lb) minced turkey (or beef)

50g (2oz) ground almonds

3 tablespoons harissa paste

1 tablespoon tomato purée (paste)

1 garlic clove, crushed

Juice of 1 lemon

1 egg

2 tablespoons extra virgin olive oil

FOR THE DIP:

200g (7oz) plain yogurt (unflavoured)

12 mint leaves, finely chopped

SERVES 4

344 calories per serving

Method

In a bowl, combine the turkey with 2 tablespoons of harissa paste, the almonds, garlic, lemon juice and egg and mix really well. Scoop portions of the mixture out with a spoon and shape into balls. Cover and refrigerate for 40 minutes. Heat the oil in a frying pan, add a tablespoon of harissa paste and tomato purée (paste) and stir. Add the meatballs and cook for 7-8 minutes, turning occasionally until thoroughly cooked.

FOR THE DIP: Combine the yogurt and mint and mix well. Skewer each meatball with a cocktail stick and serve ready to be dipped in the yogurt.

SWEET TREATS

Chocolate Muesli Bites

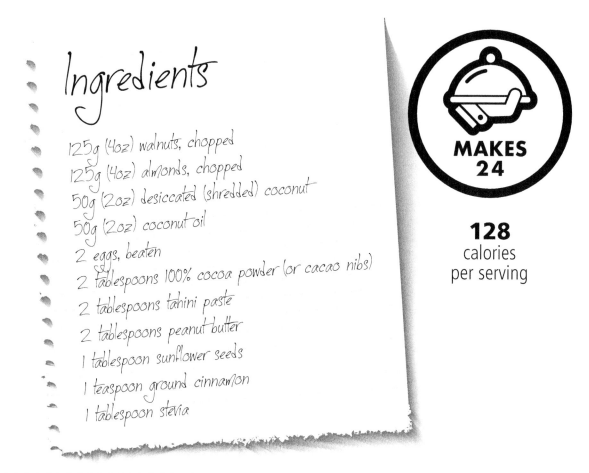

Ingredients

125g (4oz) walnuts, chopped
125g (4oz) almonds, chopped
50g (2oz) desiccated (shredded) coconut
50g (2oz) coconut oil
2 eggs, beaten
2 tablespoons 100% cocoa powder (or cacao nibs)
2 tablespoons tahini paste
2 tablespoons peanut butter
1 tablespoon sunflower seeds
1 teaspoon ground cinnamon
1 tablespoon stevia

MAKES 24

128 calories per serving

Method

Place all the ingredients into a bowl or a food processor and mix it well, keeping the nuts a nice chunky texture. Spoon the mixture into paper baking cases. Transfer them to the oven and bake at 180C/360F for 20 minutes. Allow them to cool then store them in an airtight container.

Quick Lemon Cake

Ingredients

2 tablespoons ground almonds (almond flour/almond meal)

2 tablespoons ground flax seeds (linseeds)

2 eggs

1 tablespoon butter

1 teaspoon stevia powder (or to taste)

½ teaspoon baking powder

1 tablespoon lemon juice

½ teaspoon lemon zest

SERVES 2

287
calories
per serving

Method

Place the butter in a large mug or glass dish and warm it in the microwave until melted.
Crack the eggs into the mug/dish and whisk them together with the lemon zest and juice.
Stir in the almonds, ground flax seeds (linseeds), baking powder and stevia and mix well.
Microwave the mug/dish on high for around 2 minutes or until the mixture has risen.

High Protein Chocolate Balls

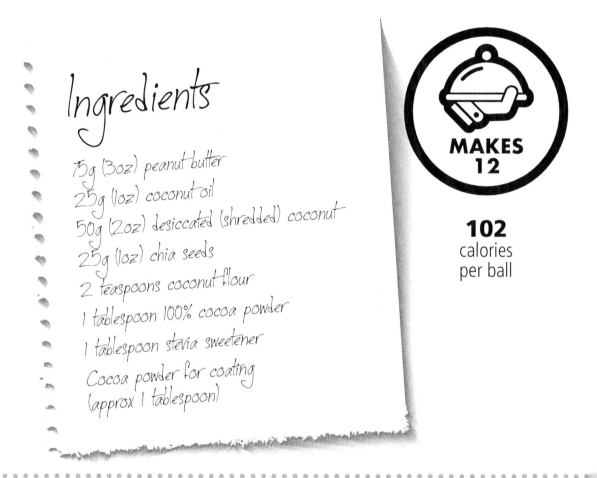

Ingredients

75g (3oz) peanut butter

25g (1oz) coconut oil

50g (2oz) desiccated (shredded) coconut

25g (1oz) chia seeds

2 teaspoons coconut flour

1 tablespoon 100% cocoa powder

1 tablespoon stevia sweetener

Cocoa powder for coating
(approx 1 tablespoon)

**MAKES
12**

102
calories
per ball

Method

Place all the ingredients into a bowl or food processor (apart from the cocoa powder for coating) and process until smooth. Using a teaspoon, scoop out a little of the mixture, shape it into a ball and roll it in cocoa powder. Chill before serving.

Pistachio Brownies

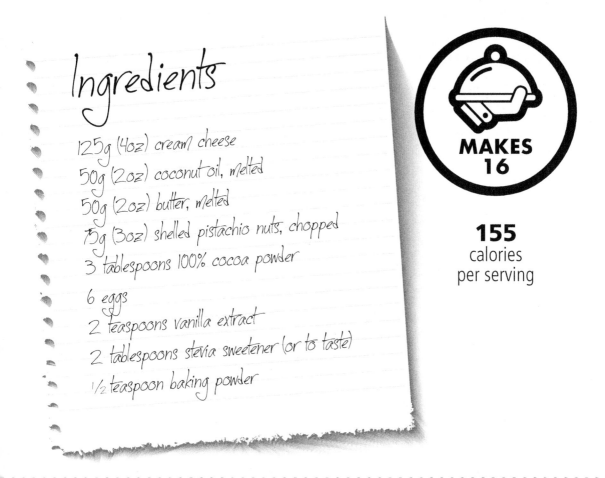

Ingredients

125g (4oz) cream cheese
50g (2oz) coconut oil, melted
50g (2oz) butter, melted
75g (3oz) shelled pistachio nuts, chopped
3 tablespoons 100% cocoa powder

6 eggs
2 teaspoons vanilla extract
2 tablespoons stevia sweetener (or to taste)
1/2 teaspoon baking powder

MAKES 16

155
calories
per serving

Method

Place all of the ingredients (except the nuts) into a bowl and combine the mixture thoroughly. Stir in the pistachio nuts. Scoop the mixture into a lined baking tray and spread it out evenly. Transfer it to the oven and bake at 180C/360F for around 20 minutes or until cooked through. Allow it to cool before slicing into portions.

Raspberry Muffins

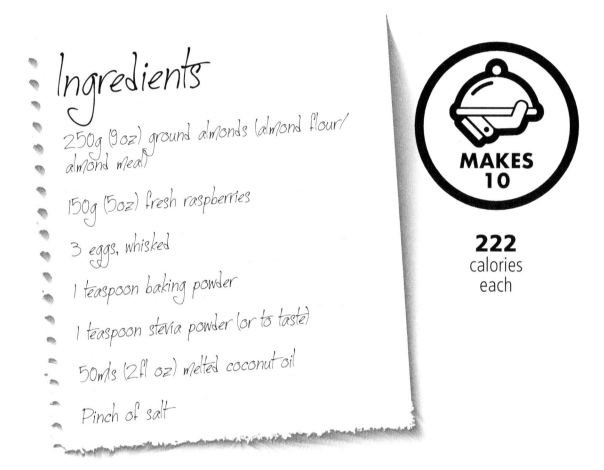

Ingredients

250g (9oz) ground almonds (almond flour/almond meal)

150g (5oz) fresh raspberries

3 eggs, whisked

1 teaspoon baking powder

1 teaspoon stevia powder (or to taste)

50mls (2fl oz) melted coconut oil

Pinch of salt

MAKES 10

222 calories each

Method

Lightly grease a 10-hole muffin tin. In a bowl, combine the ground almonds (almond flour/almond meal), baking powder, stevia and salt. In another bowl, combine the coconut oil and eggs then pour the mixture into the dry ingredients. Mix well. Add the raspberries to the mixture and gently stir them in. Spoon some of the mixture into each of the muffin moulds. Transfer them to the oven and bake at 170C/325F for around 20 minutes or until golden.

Chocolate & Pistachio Fudge Balls

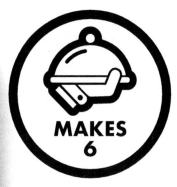

MAKES 6

80 calories each

Ingredients

125g (4oz) cream cheese (softened)

1½ tablespoons 100% cocoa powder

1 tablespoon unsalted chopped pistachio nuts

2 teaspoons stevia (or to taste)

½ teaspoon vanilla extract

Method

In a bowl, beat together the cream cheese, cocoa powder, stevia and vanilla extract until the mixture is smooth and creamy. Sprinkle in the pistachio nuts and disperse them throughout the mixture. Cover the mixture and let it chill in the fridge to firm up. Using a spoon, shape the mixture into balls. Serve chilled.

You may also be interested in other titles by
Erin Rose Publishing
which are available in both paperback and ebook.

Quick Start Guides

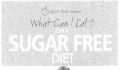
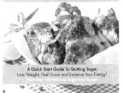
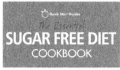
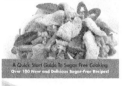
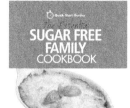
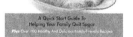
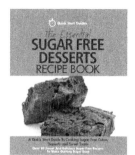
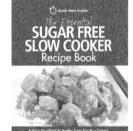
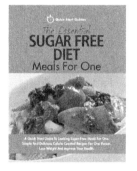
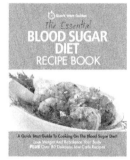
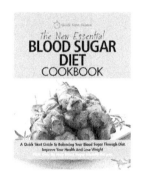
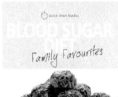
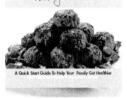
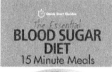
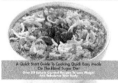
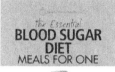
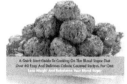
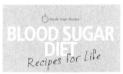
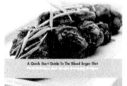
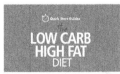
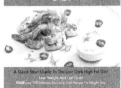
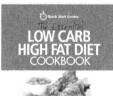
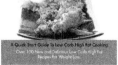
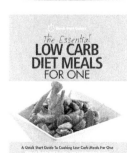
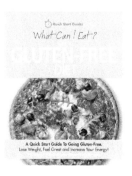

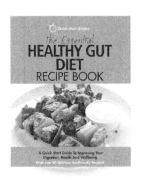
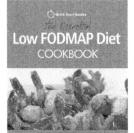
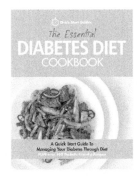
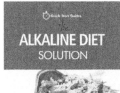
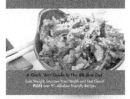
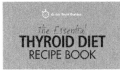
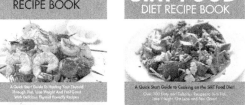
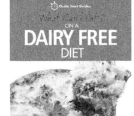
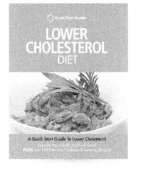
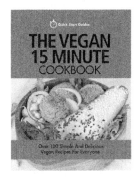
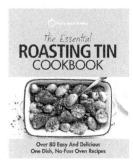
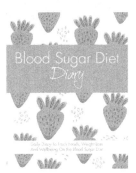
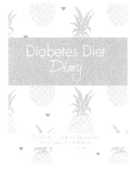
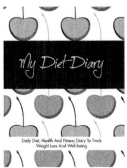
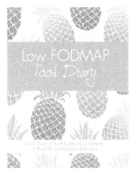
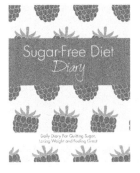
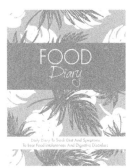

Printed in Great Britain
by Amazon

79872830R00066